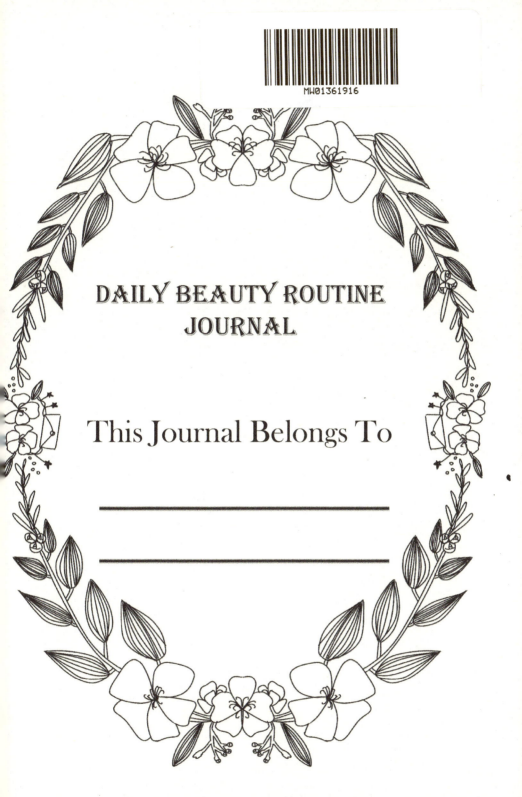

# DAILY BEAUTY ROUTINE JOURNAL

## This Journal Belongs To

_____

_____

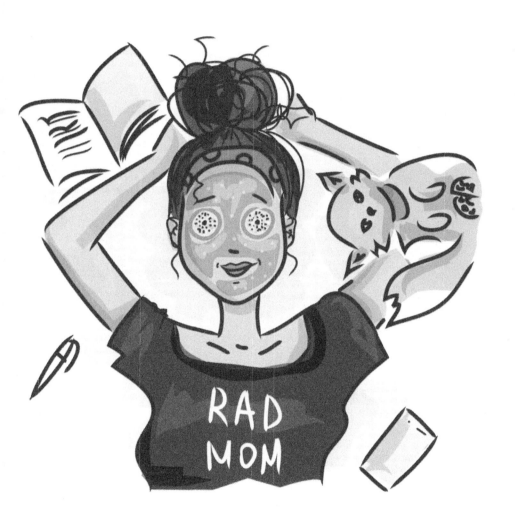

# My Morning-to-Evening Skin Care Routine

CHECK THE PRODUCTS YOU USE IN THE MORNING AND EVENING

- [ ] CLEANSING OIL
- [ ] WATER-BASED CLEANSER
- [ ] TONER
- [ ] SERUM
- [ ] MOISTURIZER
- [ ] SHEET MASK
- [ ] SUNSCREEN
- [ ] EYE CREAM
- [ ] PRIMER
- [ ] LIP BALM

- [ ] MAKEUP REMOVER
- [ ] MILD CLEANSER
- [ ] TONER
- [ ] MOISTURIZER
- [ ] EXFOLIATOR
- [ ] SERUM
- [ ] SPOT TREATMENTS
- [ ] EYE CREAM
- [ ] SHEET MASK
- [ ] NIGHT CREAM

# DAY ......

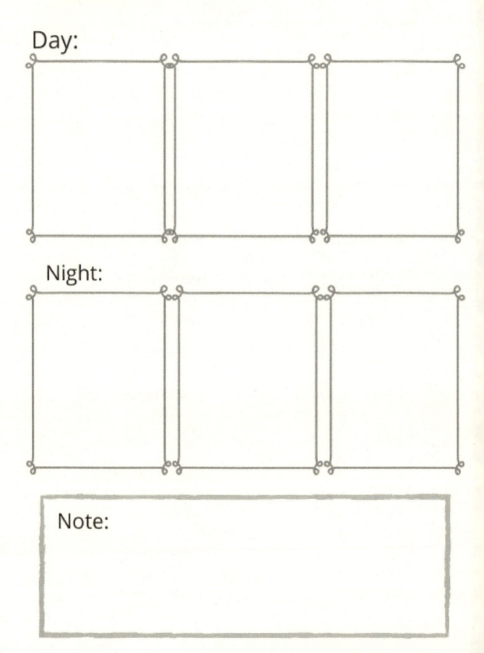

# #WAKEUPLIKETHIS

# DAY ......

Day:

Night:

Note:

# #WAKEUPLIKETHIS

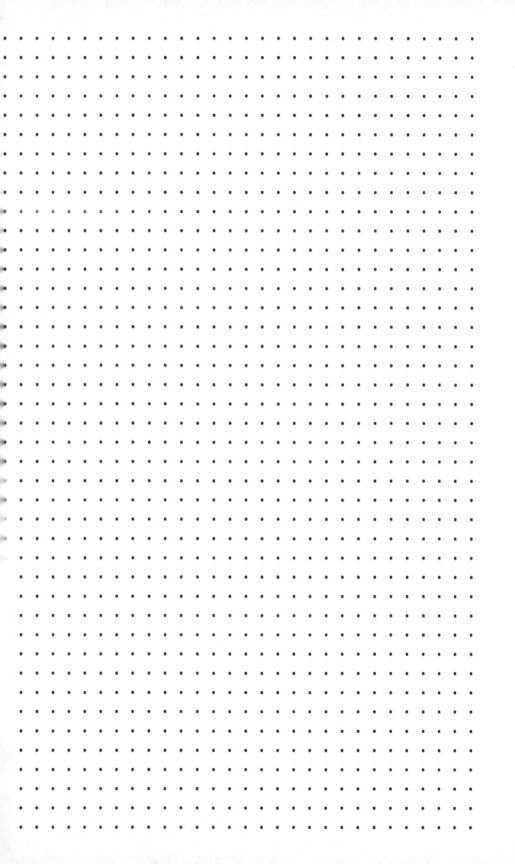

# DAY ......

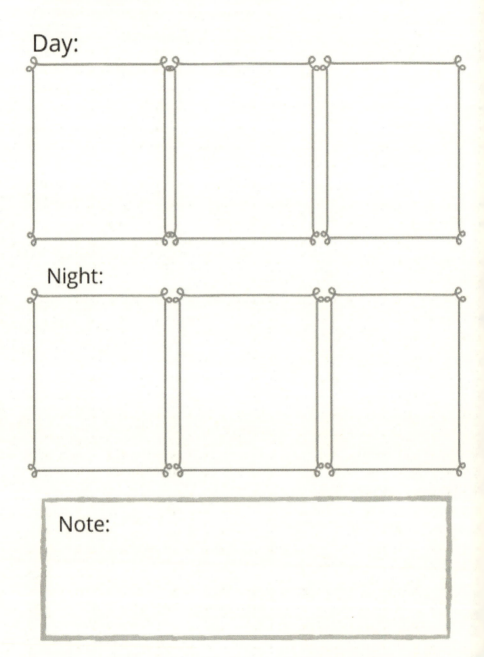

# #WAKEUPLIKETHIS

# DAY ......

Day:

Night:

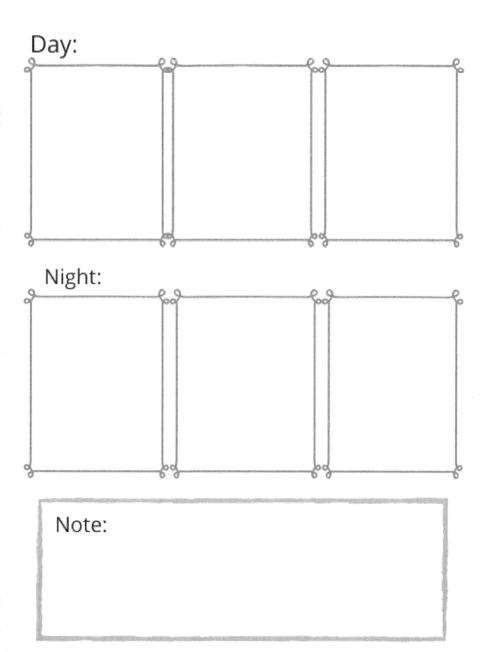

Note:

# #WAKEUPLIKETHIS

# DAY ......

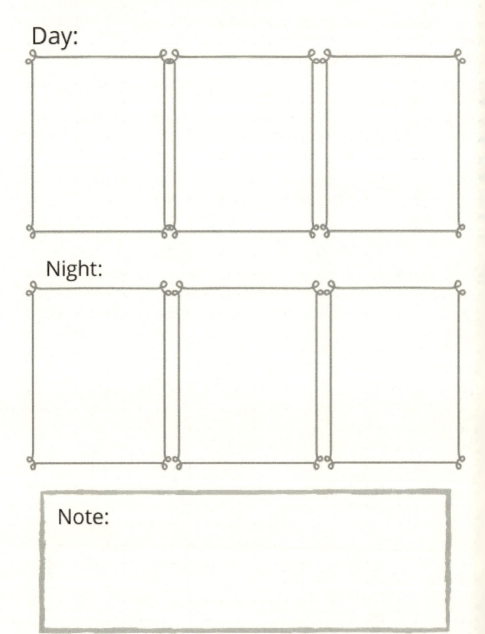

# #WAKEUPLIKETHIS

# DAY ......

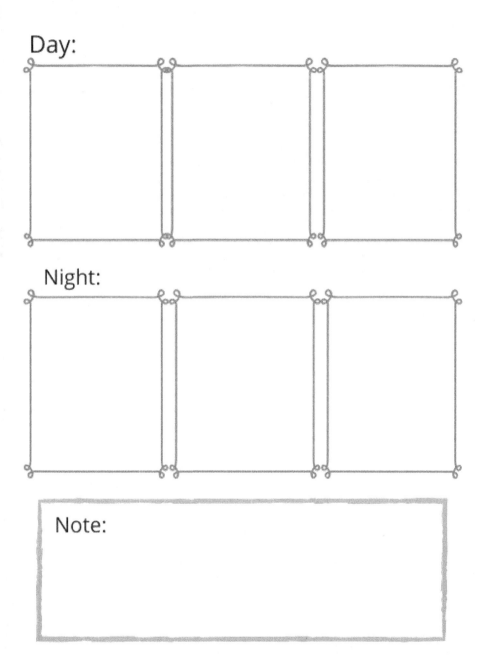

# #WAKEUPLIKETHIS

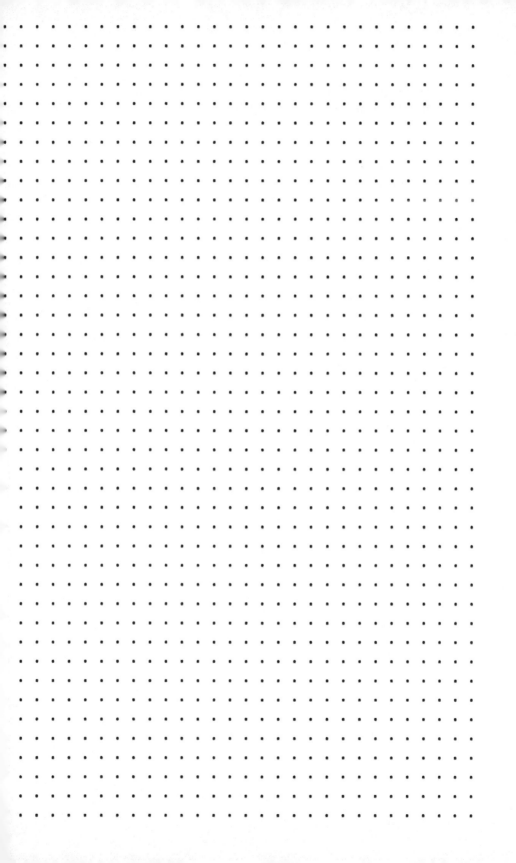

# DAY ......

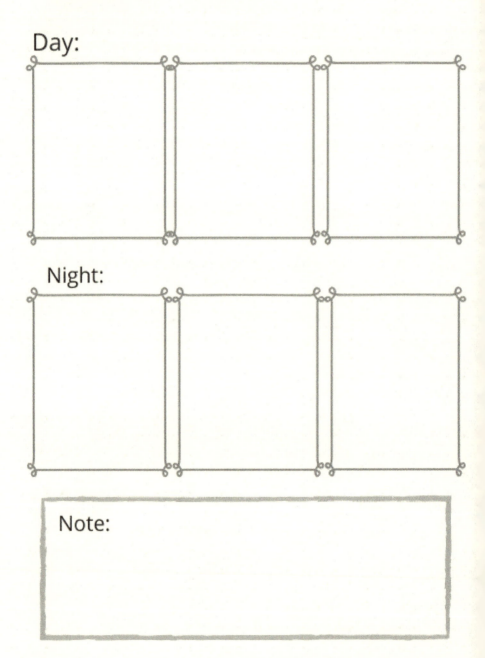

# #WAKEUPLIKETHIS

# DAY ......

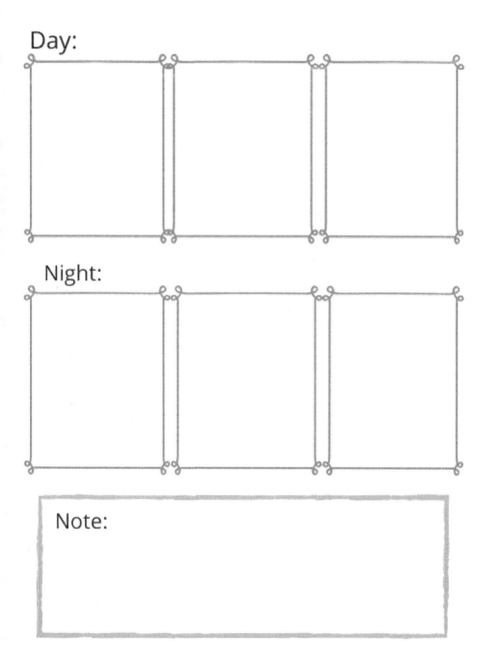

# #WAKEUPLIKETHIS

# DAY ......

Day:

Night:

Note:

# #WAKEUPLIKETHIS

# DAY ......

Day:

Night:

Note:

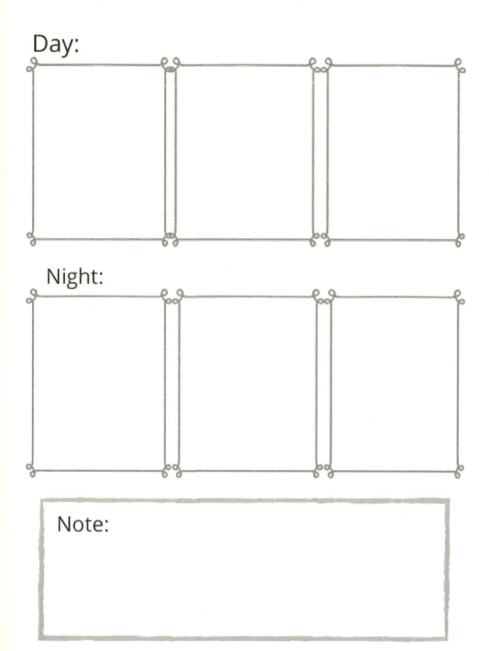

# #WAKEUPLIKETHIS

# DAY ......

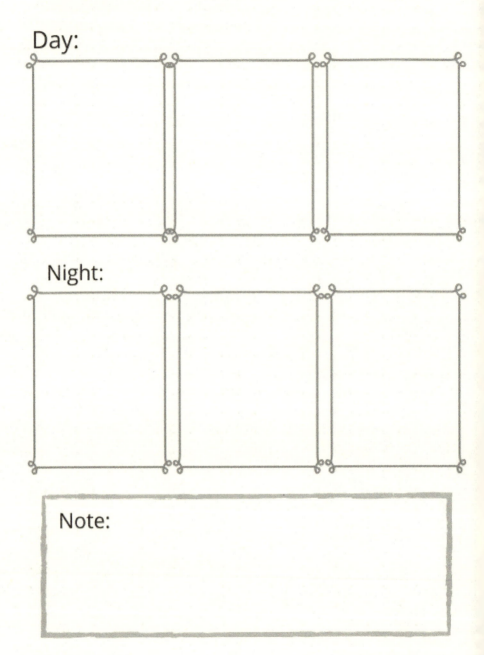

# #WAKEUPLIKETHIS

# DAY ......

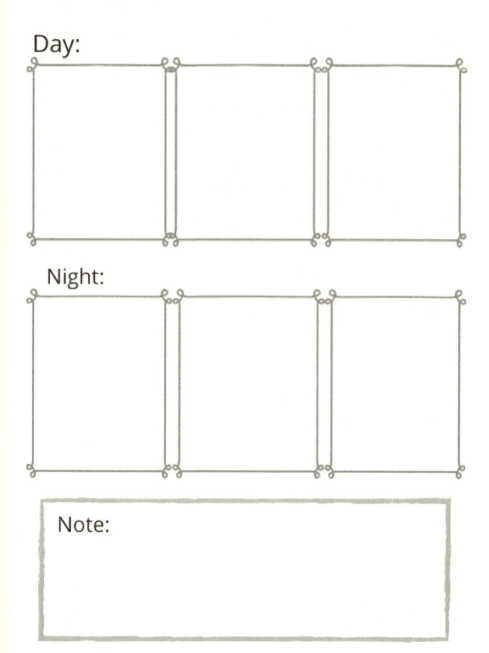

# #WAKEUPLIKETHIS

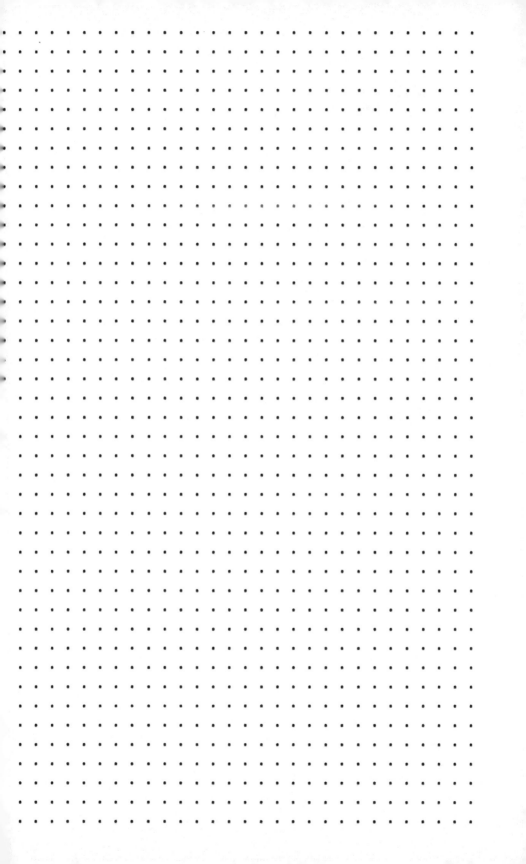

# DAY ......

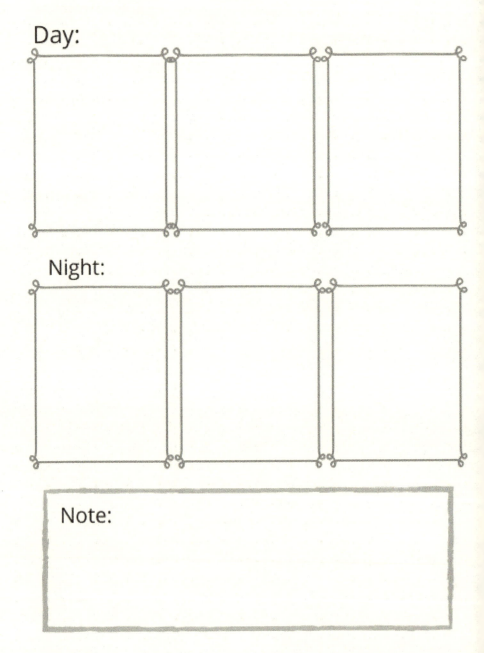

# #WAKEUPLIKETHIS

# DAY ......

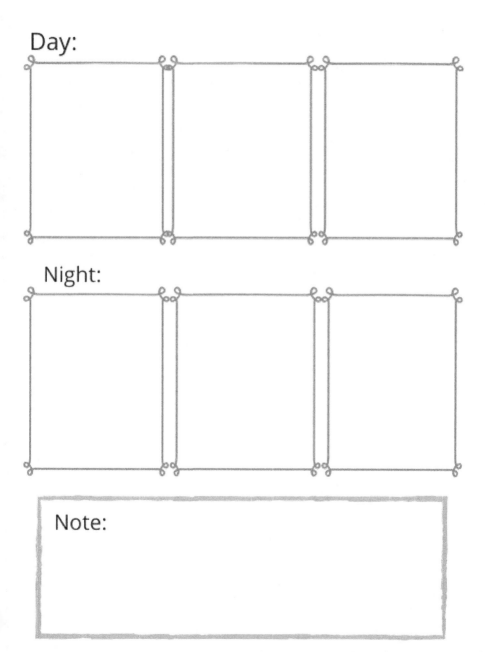

Day:

Night:

Note:

# #WAKEUPLIKETHIS

# DAY ......

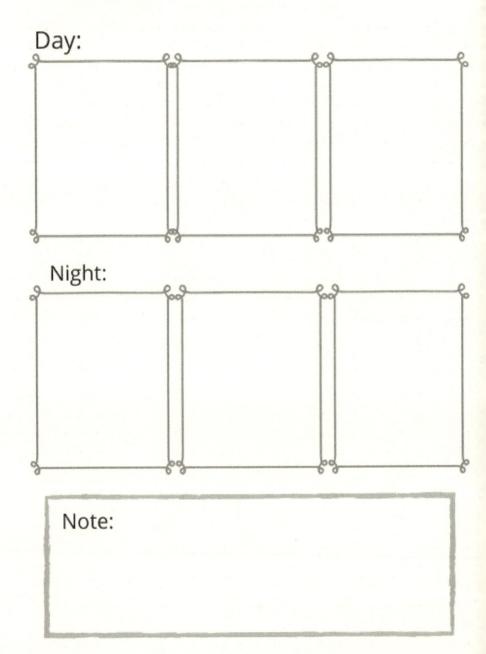

# #WAKEUPLIKETHIS

# DAY ......

Day:

Night:

Note:

# #WAKEUPLIKETHIS

# DAY ......

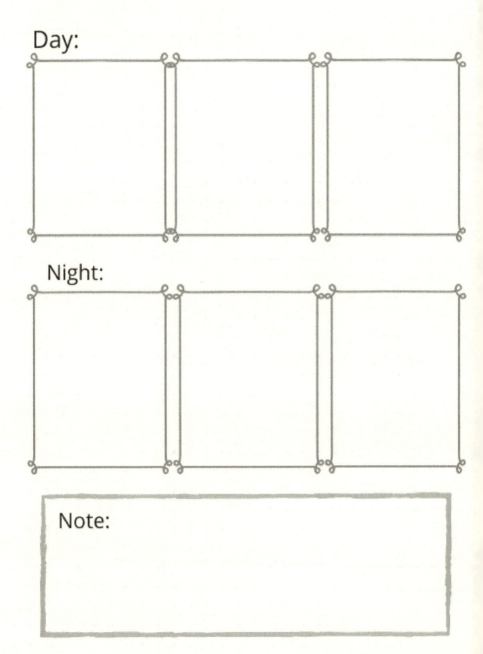

# #WAKEUPLIKETHIS

# DAY ......

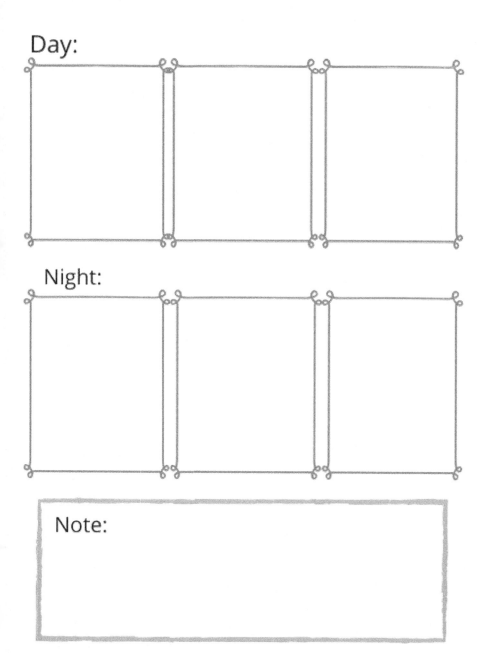

# #WAKEUPLIKETHIS

# DAY ......

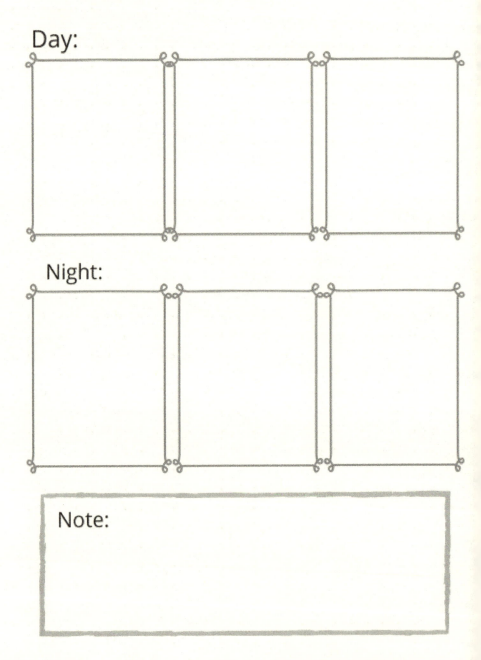

# #WAKEUPLIKETHIS

# DAY ......

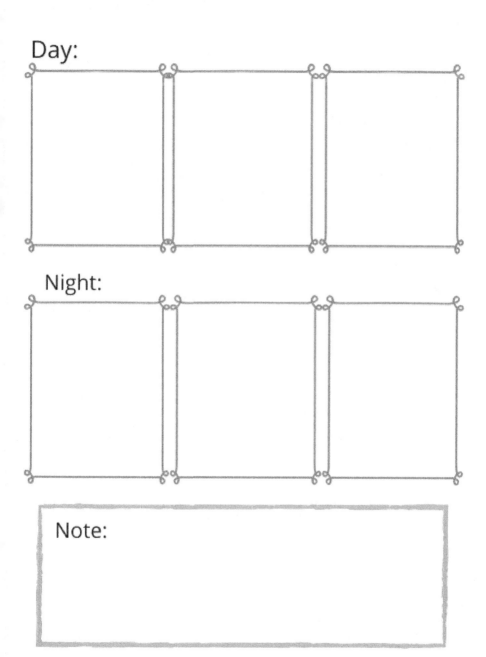

Day:

Night:

Note:

# #WAKEUPLIKETHIS

# DAY ......

Day:

Night:

Note:

# #WAKEUPLIKETHIS

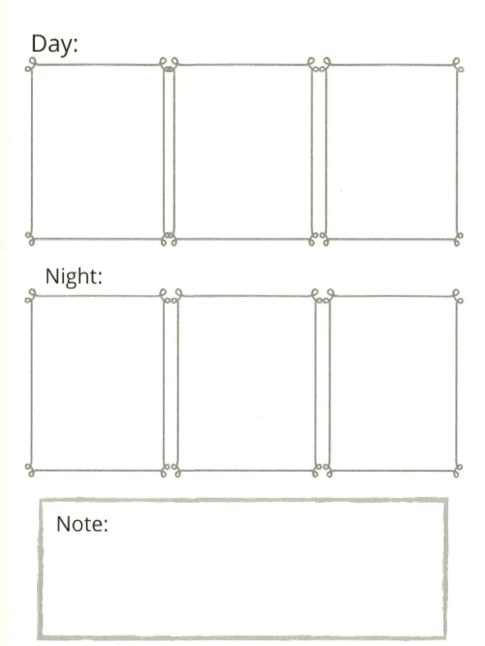

# #WAKEUPLIKETHIS

# DAY ......

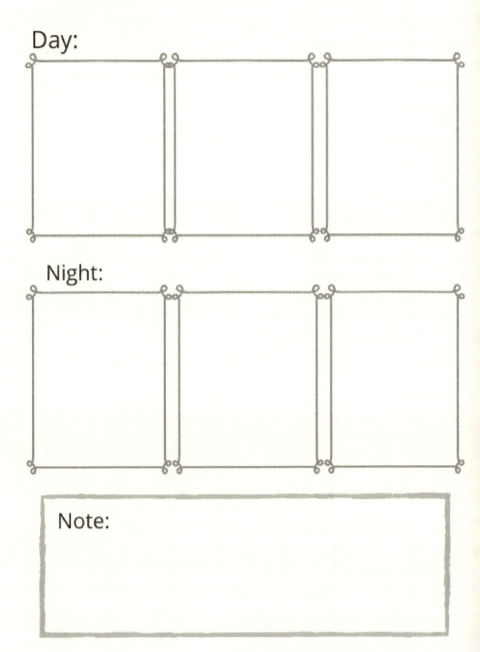

# #WAKEUPLIKETHIS

# DAY ......

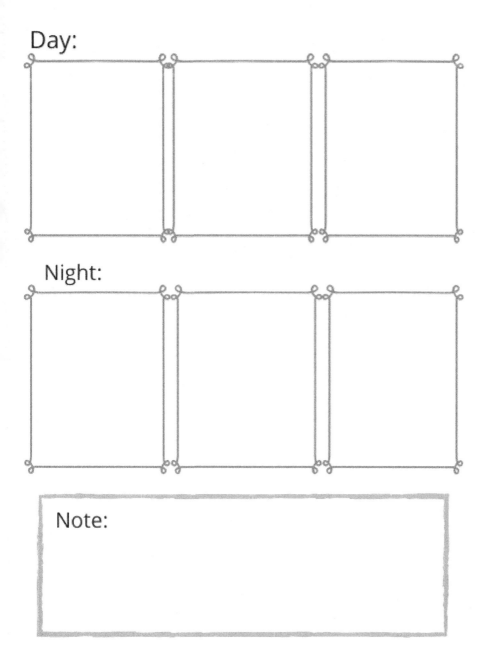

# #WAKEUPLIKETHIS

# DAY ......

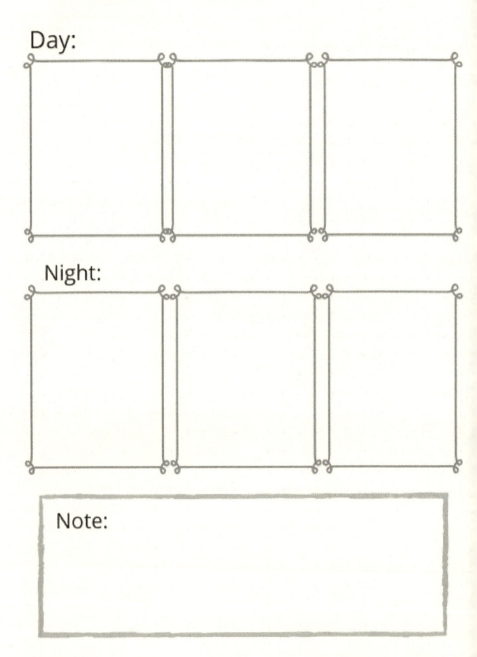

় # #WAKEUPLIKETHIS

# DAY ......

Day:

Night:

Note:

# #WAKEUPLIKETHIS

# DAY ......

Day:

Night:

Note:

# #WAKEUPLIKETHIS

# DAY ......

Day:

Night:

Note:

# #WAKEUPLIKETHIS

# DAY ......

Day:

Night:

Note:

# #WAKEUPLIKETHIS

# DAY ......

Day:

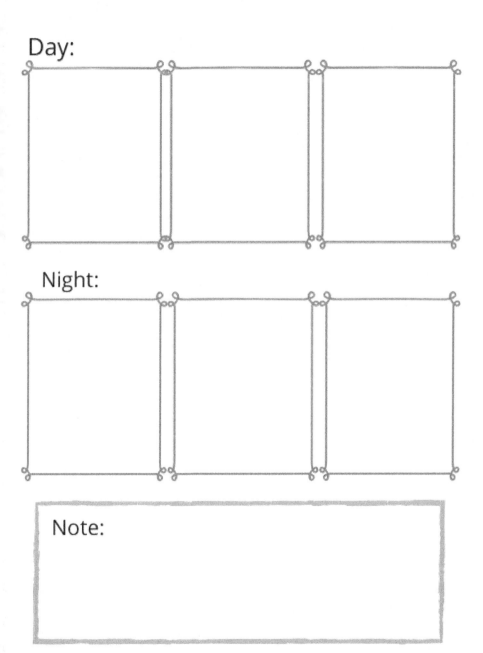

Night:

Note:

# #WAKEUPLIKETHIS

# DAY ......

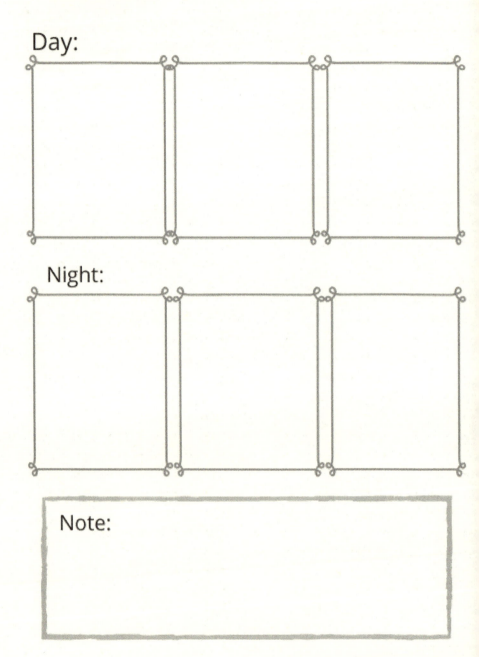

# #WAKEUPLIKETHIS

# DAY ......

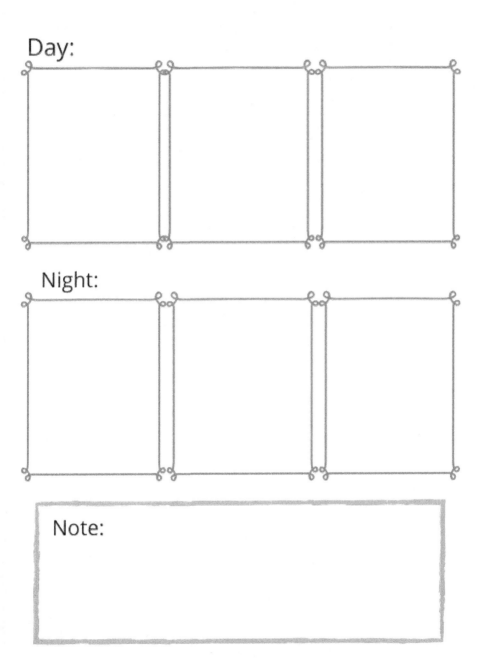

#WAKEUPLIKETHIS

# DAY ......

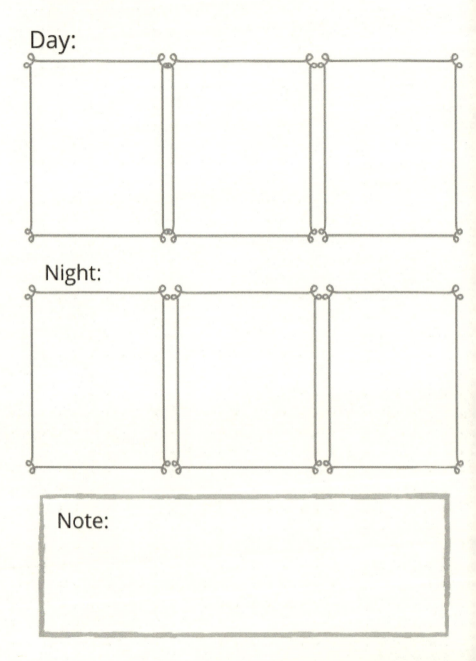

# #WAKEUPLIKETHIS

# DAY ......

Day:

Night:

Note:

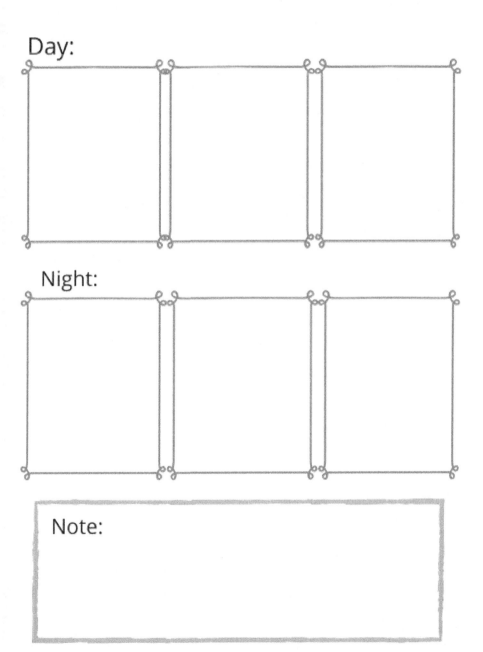

# #WAKEUPLIKETHIS

# DAY ......

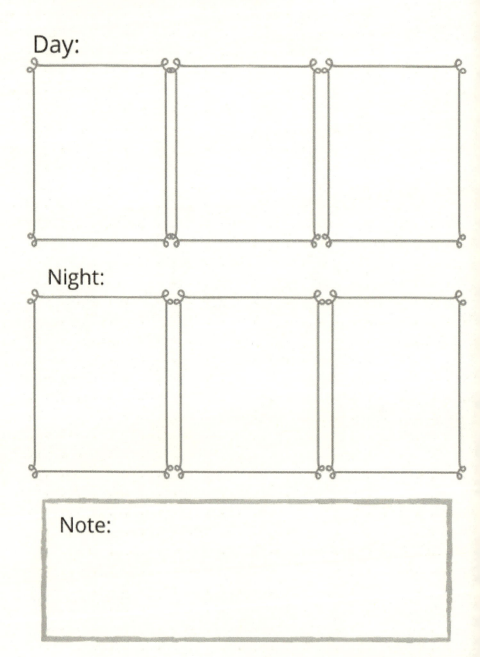

# #WAKEUPLIKETHIS

Made in the USA
Las Vegas, NV
29 April 2022